SOMETHING'S WRONG
WHEN DOCTORS DON'T HAVE THE ANSWER

LAURIE PENNER

© 2014 by Laurie Penner
All Rights Reserved.

ISBN-13: 978-1502711106
ISBN-10: 1502711109

True Story
This story is completely true, but I have disguised many of the names, except for Dr. Cory Tichauer, whose name and that of Bear Creek Clinic I am using, with permission.

Dedication
This book is dedicated to all who struggle for a diagnosis.

Contents

One 1
Two 4
Three 8
Four 11
Five 14
Six 17
Seven 21
Eight 24
Nine 28
Ten 32
Eleven 36
Twelve 39
Thirteen 43
Fourteen 47
Fifteen 51
Resources 55
Other Books by Laurie Penner 56

One

It's frightening to think you might be losing your mind.

Many times I'd experienced that strange feeling one gets when going back to work after a vacation, but this was different. When I went in to the county office where I'd been a fiscal technician for eighteen months, I felt like I'd been gone for much longer than one week. I stared at the computer screen. What was my job again?

Something was wrong with me, and it was rapidly getting worse all over. Strange shooting pains, tingling and numbness, crawling skin sensations, flaring arthritis with creaky joints, an inability to walk straight, and terrible fatigue, to name a few. The physical issues were annoying, but the mental issues were downright terrifying.

In a meeting with my boss and coworker, Nancy, after returning from my vacation, they talked about a grant project I'd been working on for six months. Then they mentioned a procedure I'd never heard of. At least, I didn't remember ever hearing of it.

I interrupted the meeting with, "Wait a minute. We need to do *what*?" Panic flooded me. *I can't do this. I don't even know what they're talking about.*

My boss explained what needed to be done, as though I could easily follow. Then he eyed me keenly. "Do you want to continue with the project, or pass it on to Nancy?"

Feeling I was mentally incapable of continuing the project, I chuckled a little. "Uh, I seem to be unable to multitask as well as I used to. I think Nancy could do a better job."

Is this what it feels like to lose your mind?

I had no choice but to wriggle out of the project, since working on it felt like certain failure. It seemed way over my head in complexity. After being able to learn many new things without a problem before, this was extremely odd. I hoped my inability to do new projects was temporary, but I figured I must be past my prime.

Walking back to my desk as though in a dream, I hoped I didn't look as crazy as I felt. I craved mediocre work that would not require much knowledge, like entering numbers on a spreadsheet. Yes, let the spreadsheet do the thinking. My brain was in some kind of walking coma.

Since my coworker had to take on my complex project, she gave me her less mentally taxing fiscal work on spreadsheets. That work I could handle. Thanking God that I was getting through the confusing day, I still found myself staring at the screen at times, wondering what I had been about to do when I looked away. Eventually I would remember, so that was a comfort. I'd heard that people who have Alzheimer's don't remember later.

My concentration had fled away at an amazing rate. When I started printing out the reports I needed in order to enter information on the spreadsheet, Nancy came over to talk.

"Are you sure you don't want two computer monitors like I have? I just look back and forth at the monitors, instead of printing out reports to go from."

Horrified, I couldn't imagine trying to hold onto information looking back and forth between monitors. "No I prefer one monitor. I think I would get... confused." Looking at various Windows on my computer was hard enough. *Wait, which one am I in? Oh yes.* I seemed unable to hold onto a number in my head while switching between windows. In fact, if I tried to hold anything in my head, I got it backwards or completely wrong.

Was it old age dyslexia? I couldn't retain the numbers unless I said them out loud, and I'd still type them wrong or have to check them again. One thing was for sure, I was working a lot slower than before. Would they still want me on this job?

Yet I could stare at a row of numbers and type them in without having to watch the computer screen. My fingers still knew how to type, even though they were stiffer. As long as I was staring at one thing at a time, I could type the information. In fact, I was getting good at staring.

My neck hurt from looking down at the desk, so I got one of those standup paper holders to keep my neck straighter. I slid the cross bar up and down to maintain my place and stared at those papers all day and typed. My boss even gave me more projects to do in spreadsheets.

I could keep working. Whew!

As long as it didn't get any worse, and I didn't make any major mistakes, I thought I might survive on the job. At times the computer monitor appeared to have a screen over it so that I squinted, which didn't help. Or did my eyes have a screen over them? That's what it felt like. My monitor was already so close that others who sat at my desk had to push it away from them.

My eyes also had an occasional involuntary tremor, which I tried to ignore. Were my eyes going bad too? Not only that, but I kept making typos. Sometimes, the typos didn't even make sense—not switched letters, but an entirely different word than what I was going to type. I had no idea why I fumbled through words so much but could type numbers accurately. I knew they were correct, because we reconciled the totals. If the numbers didn't match, we had to go back and find out why.

Was something wrong with me, or was I just getting older? The whole situation put me on edge. It felt like my ability to work was spinning out of control. At the rate I was losing mental capacity, I wondered how long I could continue. I needed to stay on the job for another year if possible, since I wasn't due to retire until the following January.

Trying not to panic, I told myself that if I could still hold a fiscal job and handle our finances at home, I must not be doing too badly. I'd been communicating normally, except for typing or saying a completely different word than the one I was thinking. Looking up the signs of dementia online didn't help. I had all the symptoms.

Whatever had hit me, it appeared to be accelerating.

Two

    By this time, many people had told me that I probably just needed more exercise for my failing body. My brother had a recumbent exercise bike that I tried out. On our vacation to Southern California, my sister also told me of her success in gaining energy with a recumbent exercise bike. Energy! That's what sold me on getting one too. It sounded like what I needed. This should help with mental health as well, right? I'd been unable to keep up a walking routine, due to being so unsteady and my legs feeling weak. Surely this was the answer to all of my health problems.

    Excited about the idea, I had started using the bike at my sister's house. The recumbent position didn't hurt my hips, which had ached for years when I sat too long on a hard surface. I'd had some kind of hip trouble for thirty years, so I padded the bike seat well. The bike seemed like the perfect way to build strength back in my weak legs without bothering my hips.

    As soon as we got home, I ordered a recumbent bike and was determined to keep it up daily no matter what. Dave assembled it for me and put it right in our tiny living room so I could peddle away during our usual movie-watching time. It was nice and quiet. If I wasn't watching a movie, I could do a word game on my Kindle. I worked up to 20 minutes a day without a problem, thinking nothing could stop me from a gradual improvement, no matter how long it might take.

    But the fatigue didn't improve, it got worse. When I tried to go for a ten-minute walk at work one day, my legs felt like they might not hold me up. That seemed not only strange but scary, since I had been working on those leg muscles.

    For weeks I noticed a growing weakness in my body but thought I'd be fine as long as I could sit down when I needed to.

Was it low blood pressure? I often felt light-headed when I stood, too. Then one day at church, even with extra padding on the chair, I was extremely uncomfortable within half an hour. My torso felt incapable of remaining upright, with aching up and down my sides.

My body wanted to lie down, so I went home and did. Why could I sit in the office chair at work and nowhere else? Maybe the small pillow behind my back helped. Sometimes I laid my head down on my desk for a minute. It wasn't just pain, but an overall discomfort that told me to rest.

A shooting pain also started coursing through my upper back at the office after a few hours of sitting. I'd been told a few years before that I had mild arthritis in my back, so I figured it was getting worse. I'd started stretching it by sitting up straight and pushing my elbows backwards, arching my neck. This released multiple creaks and pops all up and down my spine and in my neck. I was familiar with the "pop" of realignment in my back, but not with so many crackling sounds every time I did this, especially not within a few minutes of having just done it. It didn't feel like a major realignment, but a whole bunch of little ones, constantly, all day long.

Strange.

Fortunately, my car and my office chair were two places I could sit without bothering my hips too much, but I couldn't sit up straight; I had to slouch. Even in more comfortable places I squirmed constantly. I thought maybe the car seat and office chair had the proper support softness, but my pain and discomfort were getting worse, even with the exercise I was doing.

Glad we had finished extending the porch on our new house out to the driveway in the summer of 2013, I struggled up the slight incline to our car each morning. I'd pressed David the year before to get this done, because my knees didn't like going down a hill and then up nine steps to the front door.

The extended porch now leveled the walking area, so that it was level for the twenty feet going out to the driveway, and then only slightly uphill to the car. One reason I'd done this was to make it easier for my elderly parents to visit. I didn't know it would soon be essential in order for me to get out to our car and back.

Was I getting arthritis on top of the fibromyalgia syndrome? I'd been diagnosed with FMS nearly ten years before, but my fingers had gotten so stiff that I was amazed I could still type. I'd tested at about eighty words a minute when I got the job at the county office two years before, but I knew I'd slowed down. If I didn't, the words were all a jumble. As it was, I constantly had to back over a word and retype it.

Since spring was coming soon, I needed to get my vegetable garden ready, but I could barely make it outside once in awhile, much less to the garden. Our house is on the side of a hill, with uneven ground all around because we hadn't done much landscaping since building the house. I was so unsteady that it grew increasingly difficult to walk around anywhere in our yard. The garden was down a short hill about 20 feet from the house. I'd come back gasping for air. It was not like regular exercise that caused difficult breathing. More like an inability to breathe correctly. Did I have asthma? A heart problem?

My life as I'd known it was draining away, and I felt unable to keep up with everything that was getting worse, much less know what to do about it. I woke up every morning in a fog, half awake, dragging myself into the bathroom, trying to remember what I did first and hoping the rest would follow. I'd been a morning person all my life, yet now I just went through the motions. It was probably good that I couldn't hold a thought, or I would have been depressed.

At times, I amused myself with what I did, like putting a sweetener in my cup of water, but forgetting the tea bag. Later I found myself drinking sweet water. Or I would unscrew the lids off of the peanut jar and my domed snack container, pour peanuts into the snack jar, and then automatically grab the lid to put back on the peanut jar. I'd look down to find myself trying to put the snack container lid back on the peanut jar. I'd done this a few times. I would laugh but with trepidation. It was another reminder of my increasing absent-mindedness. *Well, if I start putting the ice cream in the cupboard, I'll know I'm in serious trouble!*

Meanwhile, I received a notice for jury duty.

This was another blow in a pile of issues I didn't want to deal with. There was no way I could sit in a chair or on a bench for hours throughout the day on jury duty. I needed a doctor's excuse. However, the jury summons got me started on a long trail of doctor visits that led to some answers and many more questions.

Three

I'd already received an extension on my jury duty, because my last one was scheduled during our vacation time the previous October. This time it was scheduled for February 11th, so I talked to the lady at the jury office, telling her how much pain I had when sitting. The jury office person assured me that I could stand or take a break if I needed to.

The entire jury, judge, lawyers, and everyone else in there would have to take a break because of me? Great.

Somehow, I didn't think a break would help me much at an all-day session, not to mention the mental pressure to keep sitting or standing so that the entire group didn't have to take a break because I did. The stress alone would do me in. Did they have a couch I could recline on?

Half-sitting on the couch with my head resting against the back was the only real relief from pain and fatigue that I had, other than lying in bed. On the couch, when I leaned back and pulled up my legs, I felt tremendous relief throughout my body. It took the pressure off my hips and back, plus I could rest my head. It was feeling heavier as the days went by.

In my couch position, I could prop up my laptop computer and work on my writing or go online to do research or email. I could also work on my book covers and book publishing. I was grateful to be able to do this, since I couldn't seem to do much else at home other than shuffle around the house.

Facebook was a social network I'd never appreciated while I was more active but found myself using more frequently. In writer's groups, I gradually started corresponding with more and more authors. We read each other's books, helped each other do our independent publishing, shared grammar points to remember, and prayed for each other. With little else going on other than work or reading, this kept me in touch with the land of the healthy.

I'd started getting up early in the morning, both to have more time alone for writing and to have enough time to get everything done. Having needed one hour to get ready a year ago, I now needed two hours.

Early morning proved to be useful in other ways as well. Reading the Bible first thing, God spoke comfort to me through His Word. This reassuring communication also assisted me in writing Bible study books that I wanted to publish.

I never liked going to the doctor's office, because with every visit I ended up feeling like a hypochondriac. There was invariably nothing wrong with me, or so I was told. Then one day something happened to make me realize I could no longer put off going.

I'd had heart palpitations for years, but when I felt faint at the same time my heart was racing, I realized I would have to be seen. I looked up online about tachycardia, and found that simultaneous faintness was not a good sign. One night my heart raced after I was asleep, and it woke me up, racing so much I couldn't count the beats, like some kind of electric pulse going off in my heart. It scared me.

I made an appointment with my regular doctor for February 24th and figured I'd also ask him about the heart issue, the terrible fatigue, the pain when sitting, and get out of the dread jury duty in the bargain. I'd been rescheduled a couple of times until I now had to report to the courthouse on February 25th.

I had a list of questions for the doctor, because I hadn't had insurance for so long and hadn't been there much. When I told the nurse some of my issues, I said I was "falling apart," and she laughingly said it certainly sounded like it. I hadn't even said anything about my mental state.

Doctor One was in a hurry that day, so I couldn't go into much detail. I guess I hadn't complained enough on the phone, because they had only scheduled me for fifteen minutes. When I told Doctor One about my racing heartbeat, he wanted to find a heart monitor an hour away, in Medford, Oregon, but my insurance wouldn't cover out of state. Medford was much closer than the next big city in California, because we live near the Oregon border. There was nowhere close to refer me within California.

Doctor One wouldn't let me out of jury duty but said to take pain relievers. I was devastated. Sitting there, struggling to hold my head up, I argued that I didn't want to take so many pain relievers. We'd had a friend that died from taking too much ibuprofen, plus my dad ended up in the hospital from taking it. Doctor One argued back that if he was on trial, he would rather have someone like me in the jury box than someone without the mental capabilities.

I wasn't so sure I was as mentally capable as he suggested, but I didn't say so. Maybe I should have gone in with mismatched clothes, hair askew, and drooling.

I can't do this! What do I have to say or do in order to convince a doctor that I'm not up to it?

When I went to the courthouse for jury duty the next day, I sat on my coat because of the hard seats during roll call, and held up my head by leaning my elbow on my purse in my lap. We waited about an hour in the same room, got a break, and then went back to the same room. After three hours in the roll call room they sent us home, saying to come back in a week.

I went back to the office, worked a few hours due to the jury duty I was not getting paid for and finally went home, exhausted. My hips and back were killing me, probably from sitting on the mostly hard chair and then going to work.

When I took a shower later, I noticed a small bump under my skin that was growing larger. I knew it could be an abscess, so I tried to drain it, but it wouldn't. When I developed a fever, I knew it was an infection. In bed that night my legs ached so bad that I could not rest. I took a mild codeine pill that I kept as a prescription for my cough, so I could sleep.

Calling to make an appointment the next day for a second opinion from a different physician, I still hoped to get out of the next jury duty. I wondered how truly ill people got out of it if they didn't have a doctor's notice. Maybe I could just pay a fine? I thought it would have been easier.

Four

By the time I went to my next doctor appointment, I was so ill that I couldn't believe I had ever made it to jury duty only two days earlier. I asked David to come with me so I could lean on him while walking into the clinic. I didn't feel up to driving around alone. Dave couldn't drive for me, due to a near-fatal crash while having a seizure in 2011, but he could be my moral support or help in an emergency.

With my elbow on my knee, I propped up my head once again, while I told Doctor Two about the fatigue, pain, and the growing abscess. He took a lot of notes. At least he was spending some time with me. When they took my temperature, the fever was up to 101.5 degrees. *Well, that explains a lot!*

Apparently my abscess was unusual, because Doctor Two had three more doctors in to look at it. I felt like some kind of lab specimen, while I waited for them to decide. Two of them had a discussion and almost admitted me to the hospital to drain the thing. Finally a third came in and suggested a specific antibiotic combination. Doctor Two prescribed it.

Doctor Two gave me a set of blood tests to take— a metabolic panel, among other things. He also gave me a note for one month off of jury duty. As with Doctor One, this doctor was also unsure where to send me for a heart monitor, due to my insurance coverage in California only.

Finally I was getting some help, but although I'd been there for two grueling hours, I couldn't go home yet. I had to drive us over to the pharmacy on the other side of town. David went in to get my antibiotic prescription, which was held up about an hour, due to an incorrect number or letter on my new insurance card.

I had to stay in the car and read my *Kindle* or play word games on it, while trying to recline somehow in the seat in a way that didn't hurt. I would get used to doing this, for it was to be a common position in the near future.

My infection drained by the next morning and got better, but all the commotion had taken a toll on me. I rested a few days before driving over to the courthouse so that Dave could drop off the jury note, since I was too ill to go up the courthouse steps. I couldn't believe they didn't allow me to mail it when I was so sick. You'd think being on jury duty was a matter of life or death.

When I was better, I went back to work and to the hospital afterwards for the blood draw the doctor had ordered. When the gal at the sign-in window asked for my address, I went blank. *My address....* "Um... 1321, no...1341? No...."

"Is it 1431 Bennett Drive?"

I grimaced. "Yes, that's it."

Taking a seat, I waited my turn for the blood draw, but the rest of that day was a blur. I had forgotten my own address? *What on earth?* We'd been there for twenty years!

The good news was that the antibiotic seemed to fix everything that was wrong with me. I felt great and worked hard in my garden that weekend. On Sunday morning, I was able to sing with Dave, when he led worship in church. A phenomenal change.

But the low energy and other symptoms started coming back after the antibiotic wore off. I drove home from work on March 14th, mourning my inability to do things outside in the yard. I wanted to work in my garden.

A nurse from Doctor Two's office called me at home that afternoon and said all my blood test results were normal. I felt the usual droop of defeat. How typical! The tests were always *normal*, like there was nothing wrong with me.

"Except your Vitamin B12," the nurse added. "That level is so low that it's a wonder you are able to get around. You can come down to the office right now and get a shot, if you like, and he also wants you to take a supplement. This might fix all the fatigue, racing heartbeat, and other issues you're having."

A shot. I hated shots, yet I hurried down to get it done, elated that I was not a hypochondriac.

I knew there was something wrong with me!

I'd read about a Vitamin B12 deficiency and had taken it in the past, because I so often appeared to have the symptoms: fatigue, tingling in the hands and feet, problems with balance, depression, confusion, and poor memory. Realizing I'd also started having some numbness, I could see how well the deficiency symptoms fit. I'd quit taking a B12 supplement a few years back, because one doctor didn't think it was needed if I wasn't anemic.

At Doctor Two's office, I gratefully got my injection from the nurse and was told I would need regular shots, plus an oral supplement. I was just glad the doctor had me tested and it was so easily treatable.

I got online and looked up Vitamin B12 deficiency. Poor absorption was listed as a common cause, and only about 10% of a supplement gets absorbed. That explained why supplements came in doses so much higher than what was needed. The well-known *Linus Pauling Institute* recommended that everyone over age 55 take a B12 supplement. Low stomach acid can cause less B12 to be absorbed, and I had started taking a stomach acid reducer in January. The entire B12 scenario fit all of my symptoms.

The first B12 supplement I bought turned out to have wheat in it. What? One of the reasons for a B12 deficiency was celiac disease, which I had, so I couldn't digest food if I ingested wheat. Several other common reasons for B12 deficiency had something to do with bad absorption. How ridiculous could a supplement get? It was like they'd added anti-absorption factors to the supplement on purpose. I looked for another one.

Several studies had shown that if a B12 deficiency wasn't caught within six months, the mental and neurological symptoms might never go away. Hoping mine was caught in time, I tried to find out how long it took to improve on a B12 deficiency, but all the sources just said it took several months. Some people ended up in a wheel chair or with other permanent mental or physical problems. Not a very comforting thought! My problem seemed urgent, yet I would have to wait.

Five

In my follow-up with Doctor Two, and he said my B12 level had tested at 180 picograms per milliliter, which he said was "pretty low." I'd read that "normal" was somewhere between 200 and 500, due to disagreement about such things. The doctor tried to explain to me about how B12 stays in the liver, but I couldn't follow what he said. He finished by telling me he would check the level again in two months. When I mentioned reading about B12 online, he suddenly seemed anxious to wrap up the visit and abruptly left the room.

As I was going back out through the reception area, I asked the nurse how much the shot was so I could get an idea for my budget, but the doctor came back, announced that I could just take the oral supplement, and then walked back out.

Wait a minute. What just happened?

The nurse had just told me twice that I would need a shot every week, *plus* the supplement, but now the doctor wanted me to "just take the supplement"? Was I an experiment to see if the supplement alone would work? The receptionist said something happy, like, "Oh, you don't have to have shots now!"

Yes, isn't it wonderful....?

A bit nervous, I wandered out the door to my car. Was there enough time to wait two months? What if the supplement didn't do the trick? My fatigue problem alone had kept me down for over two months, but I'd had other symptoms for months before that. Now I had to wait another two months to get the level tested again. Would the deficiency be caught in time? I didn't want any permanent symptoms. I wanted the *reliable* treatment, not the *maybe* treatment! *Can we please experiment later?*

The B12 shot seemed to help, but within one week I had extreme fatigue and mental issues again. I was sure the shot was wearing off, as they are only good for one week or less. Even the nurse had said I'd need a shot every week. It appeared that the supplement I was taking wasn't going to work like the shot had. Who knew if it was even being absorbed?

I tried to call Doctor Two, but the receptionist said he had left for the weekend. I explained I'd originally been told that I could give myself shots, so I asked them to ask him. She just said "the doctor's order is to take a supplement." Doctor Two did not call back, and it was Friday. He never did call back.

Vitamin B12 is perfectly harmless to take, so I rebelliously decided on a 1,200 mg liquid sublingual, twice a day. I felt if I took a bit more it might soak in somewhere, and I did have a little more energy right away, for a short time.

My health continued to decline overall in the next few weeks rather than improve. I woke up every day with determination to somehow carry on, trusting God to get me through. I was certain that He had a plan in all of this, and I figured one of His plans was for me to publish my new allegorical book. Maybe that was why I needed to be stuck on the couch, so I could finish and publish that book. I thought it must be a very important book for me to come under so much trouble with health.

Carrying my ideas a step further, I decided my new book would become a bestseller and support us, so we would no longer have to worry about finances. Not having to go to work sounded pretty good, although I felt a bit isolated at home, even with Dave there. We each spent our afternoons on our own computer, and Dave often had a headset on, working on a recording of either music or our pastor's sermon. And I enjoyed my job. Still, if God wanted me to write more and publish bestselling books, who was I to stand in His way?

Meanwhile, I wondered how much pain and fatigue I could endure, as both got worse. Whenever I went to rise from bed or a sitting position, my body often failed to respond the first time. My painful hips, numb legs, and stiff fingers worked with my droopy brain to convince me to stay put. Although the pain moved around to different places on my body from hour to hour, it was always somewhere, threatening me if I tempted it beyond what it felt capable of handling. One minute I could stand up and walk, and the next I tripped, staggered, or yelled "Ouch!"

Fatigue in my back caused a terrible ache after a few hours of sitting upright. My position in the office chair wasn't the problem, but all the muscles required to hold me upright felt like jelly. I often just wanted to go home and take a nap. But I had a vacation on the American Express card that I needed to pay off, so I pushed to work as many hours as possible.

I kept going to work, but it grew more difficult to maintain concentration, energy, and enough freedom from pain to stay at work. I tried pain relievers for a while, but the acidity bothered my stomach so much that by evening I had terrible heartburn. Acetaminophen worked but made me sleepy, and I was already ready to drop off throughout the day. Thankful for a kind boss, I started leaving work early, craving the comfy couch or bed, where I could rest.

David included me in his evening prayers each night for those who needed healing, as I waited for the Vitamin B12 to "kick in." I couldn't imagine going through this nightmare alone and was so grateful for Dave's tender support. He made a wonderful househusband—doing the dishes, making the bed, and continuing to make dinner every night. I wished I could afford to hire some help.

Yes, having a bestseller book would be nice.

Six

I moved as though in a time warp.

My actions slowed down, so why did the days go by faster? Entire weeks and months blurred, as though I lived in an alternate reality. The seasons hurried by before I realized they had arrived. Didn't spring just get here? Why is it almost summer?

I couldn't connect with time anymore. I used to know what happened the day before, the week before, and the month before, placing events in my life within a time period. Not anymore. Even the clock made no sense to me on occasion. 7:24 a.m. What did that mean again? Blink. Oh, I leave for work at 7:45. That's ... pretty soon. *Am I ready? No, I forgot a few things. Keep moving.*

Yet, I was never late. Nobody would know the struggle I'd been through just to figure out what time meant to me.

Enclosed in a bubble, I was the only one who knew my life was falling apart. I looked fine. I talked normally, though with hesitation. I seemed fairly functional at work and at home. But inside that bubble, something was terribly wrong with me. What could I do? Who would believe anything was amiss? Nobody but God.

Time was a blur of hours and days and weeks that hurried by, not caring that I could no longer do what I could before. But many people cared, and they prayed for me.

Concerned about becoming too self-focused, I paid more attention to others than I had before. When they asked how I was, which was way too complex to answer truthfully, I'd often say, "I'm okay, how are *you*?" In a way, I was forced out of self-focus by a simple desire to do something positive, while feeling like I was fading away inside.

I'd found an author friend on Facebook with a two-year-old daughter who had brain cancer, and I followed every post she made. One day they were a normal family with a single child, and the next day that child was being admitted to the hospital with a tumor the size of a grapefruit taking up half her brain. Dave and I both prayed for the daughter's health, which made a good turnaround a few months later. But not without those long nights and heart-wrenching days in between that tested their faith in God at every turn.

Other Facebook friends had issues as well, and I reached out whenever possible. Having published a book on Amazon, I worked on publishing more books with positive messages for those feeling trapped in various situations. I could identify.

People said things, trying to empathize with my health issues. From people my own age I usually heard, "It's hard getting old." It didn't make any sense to me, but they had no idea how I really felt. How could they? I looked fairly normal, didn't I? How would anyone know any different, unless I gave them a blow-by-blow report all day long? Who would want to hear that? Nobody.

Sometimes I would walk normally. It wasn't that bad after all, was it? Maybe I was just being a baby. Maybe I could talk myself into thinking it wasn't so bad and try to perk up and walk faster and do more. Gasping for breath or stumbling in pain within five minutes, I decided not.

There's something wrong with me. Something subtle yet debilitating. What is it?

The time approached for my follow-up B12 blood test. It was the middle of May, and I was still overly fatigued, weak, in pain, with bad concentration and getting worse every day. Thinking the B12 was probably okay by now, I asked if the blood test could include thyroid testing, and the doctor authorized it.

The blood tests showed the B12 level was up from 180 to 1500! It was very high. The thyroid test showed normal. The nurse gave me the results over the phone, and they were done.

Have a nice day.

But I wasn't done. I was still sick. Bursting into tears, I came under a huge wave of discouragement. Was all of this medical testing pointless? If it wasn't low B12 any more, or a thyroid condition, what else could it be?

After recovering, I called for an appointment again, and they gave me a physician's assistant, Doctor Three. *Hmm. Doctor Two must not have liked me for some reason.*

Doctor Three spent an hour with me, seeming very attentive and knowledgeable. I liked her. She gave me three different prescriptions, some for allergies in case that was causing the fatigue.

After I picked up the prescriptions, I read the indications that came with them. One was for depression, and it could interact with the paroxetine I was taking. I wasn't feeling especially depressed or experimental, so I took that one back, unopened.

The muscle relaxant made me depressed, so I couldn't take it either. I tried out the inhaler, but I had to imagine any improvement in my shortness of breath. The nasal spray helped with the sinus congestion I had at night, but there was no improvement in energy that I could tell. It was all a wash. Nothing worked.

Reading in my latest *Prevention* magazine that coconut oil could boost energy and was much better for you than the vegetable oils being used for the past 20-30 years, I decided to try it. We started cooking and baking with it. Coconut oil is anti-bacterial, and I'd read it could cure an infection, so I also started to eat it on the side, increasing it slowly. Maybe it would help something hiding inside of me.

At the beginning of June, I drove back to work from running an errand and suddenly felt major tingling in my left arm and numbness on the left side of my face.

Now what? Was this part of my overall condition?

Inside the office, I checked online, wondering if I needed to rush to the hospital, but it didn't appear so. I didn't have any other indications of stroke or heart attack. My racing heart had gone away with the B12 supplementation, so my heart rate had been better. Frustrated, I made yet another appointment with the doctor.

I had also noticed pain in my ear and crackling noises in my jaw, other numb spots in weird places, like the side of my stomach, or under my thigh. Pain was all over, including aching eyes, head, and... ribs.

Pain in the ribs? What the...?

My toes, ankles and back would often cramp suddenly. I kept seeing something in my peripheral vision that wasn't there after all, hearing things that weren't there, and smelling something that wasn't there. Some kind of buzzing in my ears came and went, and loud sounds often reverberated through my head, so that I had an aversion to noise or commotion in a room. Occasionally, my body temperature dropped to 97 or 96 degrees for no apparent reason. I'd go to bed hot and soon break out in chills. I only mentioned the most pressing issues to the doctor, for fear of looking like a hypochondriac again.

Doctor Three checked me over and didn't find any major back issues, so she prescribed physical therapy for the tingling. She did notice some fluid in one lung, so she prescribed an antibiotic.

Feeling sure an antibiotic would do the trick, I left happy. It hadn't escaped my notice that the antibiotic I'd taken in March had made me feel better all over. I thought I had some kind of bacterial infection still lingering that the doctors didn't know about.

But as the days went by on the new medication, nothing happened. I couldn't tell any difference from taking the antibiotic this time. I guessed it must not be an infection after all.

Seven

All I wanted in life was a bit of comfort, when I could get it. If I found a position that didn't hurt, I stayed put unless I had to move. Getting up was a difficult task I didn't want to perform. Even when my hips ached from sitting, I often just remained in the same place, squirming a bit and wanting to going back to bed. Sometimes I did, but I hated taking naps. Usually, I just turned over on the couch to rest the other side of me.

Dave began to foresee my needs, bringing me things, even without me asking at times. He made the bed every day, cooked, and cleaned when he could, though his time was often filled up with our home computer maintenance, our web site, working on sermons for the church web site, or playing guitar for the worship team. My wonderful husband gave me back and shoulder massages, even though his fingers hurt from arthritis, too.

Shuffling when I walked, I switched to tennis shoes instead of sandals, so I could balance better. I'd seen old people wearing thicker shoes. I would have limped, if I could have figured out which leg to favor. They both hurt. My hip tended to give way a bit without warning, causing me to stumble. It hurt, but then it worked again right away.

Getting in and out of the car grew difficult, especially getting out. I'd grab my cup with one hand and open the car door with the other, using the door to pull myself up onto legs that didn't feel strong. I didn't get out of the car if it wasn't necessary. When I drove Dave places, I dropped him off and went home, looking forward to my couch, where I would sink into the soft cushions and pull up my aching legs.

In the middle of June, I started the Physical Therapy with a consultation. The therapist didn't find anything in my neck or back that would cause the tingling, and I wondered what that meant. I had been certain it was some kind of pinched nerve. It was the reason I was going to PT, wasn't it? Whenever my neck and back hurt, my arm tingled, so that had to be related.

The therapist said that because I'd had the abscess in February, I'd probably gotten out of condition the past few months. I knew I was out of shape, but I'd been getting back into shape with regular exercise until the end of February, when I had the infection. After that, I felt too weak to cycle, and had fizzled on it again.

Not normally a couch potato at all, I'd worked with Dave for six years building a house and had still worked on trim and porches after we moved in. I also liked to work in the yard, when I wasn't gasping for breath every five minutes. Oh well, I would continue with the physical therapy anyway. It was all I had to go on so far, and I didn't know what was wrong with me.

A couple of days later, I had my first PT workout. I thought the tingling went away, and excitedly looked toward possible recovery. But the jaw pain and tingling came back again full force a few days later. I had a follow-up with Doctor Three on June 24th, but she just told me to keep up the PT and come back when I was done. The ladies in the doctor's office cheered when I didn't need another appointment, as though that meant I was all better now.

Oh yeah, I'm just great.

My back and neck along the spine had grown especially painful at work. I was trying to keep up six hours a day at the office but often went home early or skipped an entire day. Walking turned into a precarious feat of balance and pain. I had thought about getting a cane so I wouldn't fall, but instead I just walked slower, putting one foot carefully in front of the other.

My mental state had not improved on the B12 as I'd hoped. My concentration was so bad that it was a wonder I could still do my job. My coworker noted things that I forgot a couple of times, things that sounded completely unfamiliar. I couldn't believe the difference in my memory.

Tremors plagued my feet and hands. I couldn't seem to hold my feet still. When I wrote something, the pen seemed to have a mind of its own in my hand. I wasn't sure if this was my hand not working right, or my head.

Searching online didn't help much. With so many symptoms, I began to enter several at once to see if some strange disease fit, but I kept coming to a dead end.

One day, a co-worker heard about my symptoms and sent me a podcast interview with a Lyme disease specialist at the Bear Creek Naturopathic Clinic in Medford. I had looked up Lyme disease before and found that I had almost all the symptoms. However, I didn't remember getting bit by a tick, and I'd had no rash. I'd had ticks on me before, and figured I would know if I'd been bit by one, especially if it had remained attached.

When I kept reading, I found out the tick bite and rash were often overlooked by a Lyme victim, and the truth sank in. Only half the victims got a rash, and if the tick was a nymph, it could be no larger than a poppy seed. Once I'd noticed a bloody spot in my ear, with a tiny black speck in it. Then it hit me— the little black spot in my ear could have been a nymph tick!

Wow. I could have Lyme disease.

Eight

Lyme disease is caused by a *spirochete*, a bacteria especially good at avoiding both testing and treatment. I watched the video *Under Our Skin* and saw how bad the disease could get if left untreated. The spirochete invaded not only the joints, but the heart and brain.

The statistics show that the standard test for Lyme disease has been especially inept at detecting it, especially after several months have gone by.[1] It was designed to be done on patients who got bit by a tick a few weeks earlier. It will not detect antibodies if done too soon, but it also doesn't work well if done too late, because after some time antibodies do not detect the Lyme bacteria that are hidden in tissues by this time. However, because the Center of Disease Control has continued to recommend doing this test before other tests, most doctors do no not think the patient has Lyme. A lot of people have slipped by undiagnosed.

Far from being a senior citizen disorder, Lyme disease was first discovered in Lyme, Connecticut, when researchers investigated why so many children were getting diagnosed with juvenile arthritis. *Under Our Skin* showed young people scooting around on the floor to get somewhere in their house, screaming in pain, crippled, paralyzed, or barely able to move. Some were very young but ended up in a wheel chair or with a heart attack or dementia. A few have died.

Could these young people have been helped sooner and led normal lives if only medical practitioners were better informed? Then why aren't they?

---

[1] www.ILADS.org http://lymedisease.org, http://sheamedical.com/lyme-disease, http://canlyme.com to name a few.

In one study, research done on deceased Alzheimer's patients indicated the presence of Lyme bacteria in 7 out of 10 brain samples. [2] *A lot of Alzheimer's cases could be prevented?*

No wonder I identified so much with the symptoms of Alzheimer's.

People told their stories of misdiagnosis: fibromyalgia (FMS), chronic fatigue syndrome, multiple sclerosis, Parkinson's disease, and mental illness. Lyme disease is often called the "great imitator." When diagnosed at a late stage— months or even years after infection— some Lyme victims have gone on antibiotics for months or even years, unable to tell for weeks or months at a time whether they were getting better. The expense left them bankrupt. Many were suicidal. The suffering involved was staggering.

The ninety-minute video *Under Our Skin* was depressing to me. Suddenly, I wasn't sure Lyme disease was better than a brain tumor. At least that might be cured sooner and maybe cheaper. Whatever I had, I needed a diagnosis as soon as possible. Letting it go on too long was certain misery or worse.

Since we live on the edge of a forest where deer wander all over our yard, ticks are abundantly available, but when I looked online, I saw that our county reported only a few Lyme disease cases a year. It seemed highly unlikely that I could have Lyme disease, yet what was happening in my body matched every symptom list on each web site I investigated, including some of the most absurd symptoms I'd ever heard of.

One of the symptoms was the feeling of something crawling on my skin, like a spider, when nothing was there. This happened so often that I got used to it. It was just one of the many issues I had. One day I felt something on my arm and looked down to see a tick crawling on me. You should have seen me jump and fling that thing into the air! Fortunately, Dave found it right away. *Whew! Is that a sign of what I have?*

When I found out that Lyme disease was easily eradicated if caught within a few months, I realized I was rapidly approaching the last boundary of a simple treatment. It had been six months

---

[2] http://bebrainfit.com/lifestyle/drains/lyme-disease-a-hidden-cause-of-mental-decline-and-alzheimers

since my worst symptoms started showing up in January. If something wasn't done soon, I could end up with late-stage Lyme disease, and it didn't sound pretty.

Was I being unreasonable? What if my mental processes went downhill before I could get help? My family didn't know any more about Lyme disease than the average person, though I'd started to talk about it all the time. They probably chalked it up to hypochondria and considered me paranoid, which is ironically yet another symptom of Lyme disease. But I was the only one who knew something was wrong with me. If I was going to get to the bottom of this thing, I'd better do something... *NOW*.

In a leap of faith, on July 2nd, I made an appointment at the Bear Creek Clinic, per the podcast I'd heard. Called an LLMD for Lyme Literate Medical Doctor, this kind of doctor specializes in Lyme disease. The receptionist said that Dr. Cory only treated Lyme victims now, but I couldn't get in until August 29th, eight weeks away. Due to so few Lyme doctors in the area, he was overwhelmed with patients. While still on the phone, a wonderful idea hit my brain, surely from God Himself. I asked to be on the cancellation list.

When I got off the phone, I sent out an email request to friends and family, asking them to pray for a cancellation so I could get an earlier appointment. My insurance wouldn't cover it, but this doctor was only an hour away, and I suddenly didn't care what the cost was. Putting it on a credit card, I would pay it back later. My health had become way too important to ignore any longer.[3]

Determined to work on Doctor Three to get tested for Lyme disease while I waited for my Bear Creek appointment, I dropped off a list of my Lyme symptoms at her office on Monday afternoon, asking her to call me. When she called back, I explained my concerns, pointing out how the antibiotic in March had helped me so much. I told her I didn't remember a tick bite, but something in my ear produced blood with a black spot, which could have been a

---

[3] I later chatted with people who went through this same type of experience or worse. One lady said her LLMD was almost three hours away. One man said he'd come from Iceland to the U.S. to get help.

nymph tick. She agreed to do the test, but her final response sounded like a well-rehearsed line: "Please be assured there is no prevalence of Lyme disease in this county."

Interesting response, but better than some receive. A friend said a doctor informed her in no uncertain terms that there was no Lyme disease in California. Others said their doctors told them Lyme disease wasn't in Siskiyou County. I wondered why, since I'd seen online that at least a few cases in our area had been reported to Public Health. Did our Public Health not communicate with the doctors? I also found out there is a vaccine for Lyme disease for dogs in our county. Are they more concerned about dogs than people? Or are the veterinarians better advised?

Doctor Three also ordered testing for autoimmune disorders like Lupus and rheumatoid arthritis, for which I was grateful. I dreaded a diagnosis of just chronic fatigue syndrome because there was no cure. My sister had been through that before, and it was awful. But my oddball symptoms had gone beyond just extreme tiredness. It had to be something more.

Relieved that I was finally getting checked for more issues, I went to my PT appointment. When I told my therapist about my scheduled time in Oregon to check for Lyme and the local doctor testing it as well, he was intrigued. He said to be sure to keep the appointment in Oregon, no matter what the test showed. His wife had a tick bite once and even the characteristic bull's eye rash, but the local doctor wouldn't test for Lyme. He said it "wasn't prevalent in Siskiyou County." Hmm. I'd heard that before!

Yet here was an example of someone else in our county who had gotten Lyme disease, trying to get treatment, and getting turned away.

Why do the doctors keep saying it isn't here?

After that, the more people I talked to, the more I found who either had Lyme disease or knew someone who had, right there in Siskiyou County.

Nine

By the time I'd researched more about Lyme disease, I expected a negative test. If I had Lyme, I'd already had it too long to get an accurate result. I'd been educated. The spirochetes can encapsulate to protect themselves from antibodies, so they need to be drawn out into the bodily fluids, where the antibodies will show up on the test. This can be done by starting antibiotic or herbal treatment a couple of weeks before testing. It brings them out of hiding.

Research organizations have documented thousands of cases where someone's Lyme test has indicated a false negative.[4] How did they know they were false? Because a properly done test will eventually show positive, if the doctor knows what he's doing. The CDC web site makes it sound worse to get a false positive than a false negative. Their site refers to a report from 1994, where even the site itself says it "might be outdated" because it's twenty years old.[5]

No wonder so many people have had to do their own research!

An unknown number of patients have remained untreated until they were so overcome with Lyme bacteria that they were much harder to diagnose. Just getting a diagnosis sounded like a huge mountain for too many people in the overall treatment for Lyme disease, and as many as 25% of Lyme victims have been

---

[4]Compare CDC guidelines as of September 21, 2014:
http://www.cdc.gov/lyme/diagnosistesting/LabTest/TwoStep/index.html with www.ILADS.org, http://lymedisease.org, http://sheamedical.com/lyme-disease, http://canlyme.com, http://lymedisease.org/news/lymepolicywonk/lymepolicywonk-the-lyme-wars-guidelines-controversy-and-informed-consent.html

[5]http://www.cdc.gov/lyme/diagnosistesting/LabTest/TwoStep
http://www.cdc.gov/mmwr/preview/mmwrhtml/00038469.htm

children![6] *Would somebody please wake up the medical community?*

Some doctors with compassion have decided to treat their patients with antibiotics, based on a clinical diagnosis. Several have lost their license to practice, even as their patients got better. This has led to years of battles between the CDC and the research groups: The "Lyme Wars."[7] Others have reverted to natural cures to avoid the medical field and the fighting. Herbs don't usually harm anyone, but they can just as easily get rid of the bacteria, by providing an unfit environment in the body for them to live.

In my case, sure enough, the doctor's office called me and said all my tests were negative. I almost laughed. To the doctor, that meant no Lupus, no Rheumatoid Arthritis, and no Lyme. What I'd researched was coming true before my eyes. I was turning into a classic case of a Lyme victim that gets ignored! It wouldn't stop me from continuing to seek help, no matter what they said. I merely asked how to get copies of my test results so I could show the doctor at Bear Creek Clinic.

The receptionist told me my doctor's instructions— to continue the physical therapy and then come back, if needed. *Right. Get more exercise somehow, when I can barely shuffle around a room or sit on any surface.* Even my physical therapist had seemed skittish about having me do too much. I wasn't sure if I should be exercising or not.

I'm steadily getting worse, and the only one that knows something's wrong is me. If my brain deteriorates enough, pretty soon I won't know either.

The date at Bear Creek was weeks away, and time wasn't rushing by for me like it had been. It seemed my appointment would never get here as I labored through each work day. Sitting in one place grew harder, as I squirmed in my office chair, wondering how silly I looked. My fatigue grew worse, and pain struck in my hips, shoulders, neck, and back at odd moments.

After four hours at the office desk, I went home exhausted. I took a nap every day after work, to replenish my energy and relax

---

[6] http://originsofhealth.com/articles/get-educated-about-lyme-disease
[7] http://www.sheamedical.com/the-battle-for-the-truth-about-lyme-disease

the strain of holding myself upright. It helped, though many times I didn't want to get up again. I'd shuffle out to the couch and sit, staring at the coffee table. As I reclined on the couch before Dave made dinner, I'd pick up my laptop and get on Facebook, mostly to have something easy enough to do.

To get an idea of how difficult this is, picture how you feel when you're coming down with a bad cold that includes a low fever. You know that "low-energy" feeling, where your body is trying to tell you to rest? You might rest or you might keep going, depending on how bad you feel. You might be able to continue working every day, but it's hard. Now imagine going through that low-energy feeling without letup every day for weeks and weeks.

That's how it feels. You got it.

A fellow author who knew I was being tested for Lyme posted a suspense novel she had found on my page. The main character was a middle-aged woman with Lyme disease. I eagerly bought the e-book. I found *Over the Edge* by Brandilyn Collins not only well-written but highly informative. The main symptoms the character described in the book were similar to mine, and I could identify with this character, because no one believed she could know more than the medical establishment that tested her. I sent an email to Brandilyn, and she wrote back words of encouragement, because she'd had Lyme disease herself. Twice.

In further research online, I came across a web site where a woman claimed that coconut oil cured her of Lyme disease. That sounded good! I was still using that in cooking and eating it, but I increased the amount, wondering what else I could do toward wellness, while waiting to be seen by Dr. Cory at Bear Creek Clinic.

When I checked around for more about the natural healing of Lyme disease, I came across a web site recommended often by other sites. A man named Stephen Buhner had written *Healing Lyme*, a book about the curing of Lyme disease using herbs. Since the book wasn't expensive I ordered one, hoping to get started on some of those herbs.

My own new allegorical book that I'd published in March was not only selling poorly, my other book sales were dwindling also. I'd self-published a few Bible studies, but I had no mental organization to market them. *So much for bringing in more income with a bestseller.* My life seemed to be on hold, and my usual hobbies and interests reflected my illness. Though Dave had helped me keep the garden going, it produced a mere handful of anything all summer. Just like me, it sat there soaking up water but not giving anything back. Two of my five indoor plants had died or were dying. You'd think I'd infected my plants as well.

My quilting had gone by the wayside, as had my guitar-playing, which hurt my fingers and back. I hadn't been able to sing with Dave to lead the worship at church. The trim inside our house had never been finished since that was my forte. The tile we'd bought for our kitchen counter still sat in boxes on the front porch a year after we bought it, because we needed to work on the installation together. Dave had worked on extending our porch the other direction over the summer, so that the roof over it would shade the west side too. I wanted to help build it, but I couldn't.

All that was left was my reading and writing, although trying to follow a long sentence was becoming impossible. I couldn't hold the thought at the beginning of the sentence past the next phrase, so I had to read the sentence over and over. It was probably good mental exercise, but I often never grasped the meaning of the sentence, even after several tries.

I'd hoped to start an editing business some day, because several authors enjoyed my editing style, but I needed a better brain for that. One needed to watch for continuity, and my sense of timing had disappeared. I could still write, but it was disorganized. I kept forgetting where the story was chronologically and had to label each scene by the day of the week and the time of day so I could see if it was in order. When I did that, I discovered several places where events were out of place with each other.

Social Security retirement began to look like the only viable income option for me. I hoped my remaining years weren't going to be in bed.

Ten

A lot of friends and family on my email list or on Facebook kept praying for me. One night a couple from church came by to pray for me in person. Our pastor prayed for me at church, when I dropped Dave off or over the phone. Grateful for all the prayers, I continually thanked God for all of these people who cared enough to follow my health issue.

Meanwhile, our finances were in question. Since it was so hard to sit at my office desk for six hours, I began to take a lunch break in the middle. Curling up in the car relieved my hips and back somewhat, and I could read my *Kindle* during lunch. That helped for a while, but by the second week in July I couldn't keep working that many hours. At the same time, we now had lots of medical copayments coming due, on top of our regular bills. My insurance copayment was $40, and it appeared on bills coming in from several doctors, labs, physical therapy, and testing facilities. Dave and I prayed for a financial answer.

It dawned on me that Dave's mother might be willing to help our daughter Becky in her final year of college. Becky worked at a hospital almost four hours north of Medford as part of earning her degree from the Oregon Institute of Technology to be a nuclear medical technician. Within two days of asking, Becky's grandma agreed to support Becky in our place, relieving our bills by several hundred dollars a month. My wonderful boss also agreed to let me cut back my work time to only four hours a day. *What a relief!*

Yet, other financial issues plagued me.

When Dave had surgery for a brain abscess in 2000, he had lost much of his short term memory, so I'd been taking care of the finances. Dave's Social Security income, his small monthly VA stipend, my paychecks, and my forty dollars per month in book royalties were all set up as automatic deposits, so I wouldn't have to run to the bank all the time. I kept track of the bills and income on a computer spreadsheet program. Working on a spreadsheet was my specialty. It was how I'd gotten my current job. But I began to see more math errors when balancing the checkbook, and they were mostly mine.

One day I discovered I hadn't listed one of our credit card bills on my home budget, a $200 payment. I had forgotten about it, and it was due in two days. How could I forget such a thing? Only by God's grace could we pay the bill and get it done in time. Setting up every possible bill as an automatic debit from the bank, I hoped I didn't also forget to subtract something from the checkbook register.

We used a bank debit card, but keeping track of Dave's debits had become sporadic. He couldn't remember to give them to me, and I couldn't remember to ask him. I was even forgetting my own debits. I had to look up our debits on our online bank account all the time. Often I forgot to balance the checkbook and was aghast at my lack of monitoring. If neither one of us could remember to track our debits and bills, what kind of financial mess would we make? I'd heard of people in their eighties or nineties having this problem, but we were still in our sixties. *God help us!*

I wasn't used to this! I could remember holding all this information in my head before, accounting for the bills that were coming due and even how much we owed. Now I could barely track it on a spreadsheet. I could only hope that God would hold it all together for us. Our bills had turned into mere numbers, instead of having more meaning in my head. They either added up or they didn't. The reasons for discrepancy could be mysterious, although I managed to balance our account once in a while, even with errors. As at work, I had to proceed by rote at home. On each payday we paid certain bills, so they got paid. If they weren't on the budget they got ignored. I entered all debits into a spreadsheet to account for any math errors in the checkbook, but I constantly got lost trying to use spreadsheet formulas if I had to figure them out.

We lost bills, too. Dave and I both lost a car registration that came in the mail, and I couldn't remember seeing it in the first place.

"Are you sure we got a bill?" I asked him. "Do you remember if it was due yet?" Dave requested another form online, but we were looking all over the house for days and in the same places. I prayed to find it and looked in an odd place. *There it is!*

Our finances felt out of control, and so did my brain.

To make financial matters worse, my medical appointment at Bear Creek Clinic was outside of my insurance coverage. That meant all costs had to come out of pocket. I had not been able to find a local Lyme Literate Doctor. The closest LLMD to us in California was in Chico, according to a handy online Lyme doctor directory. Chico was nearly three hours away. A friend recommended a naturopathic doctor in Redding, just a ninety-minute drive, but I wasn't convinced he knew a lot about Lyme disease, and it still sounded too far to drive. My body didn't handle a thirty-minute trip well, so I didn't think it would handle a ninety-minute one.

My legs or feet would cramp when I drove very far though, and sitting upright was difficult. Once I was driving on a small canyon road and got a foot cramp that wouldn't dissipate. Since we were almost to our destination, I didn't want to stop. I usually put the car in cruise control on the freeway whenever I could so I wouldn't have to hold my foot down. My foot kept cramping, so I tried cruise control at 25 mph. It worked! Amazed it would hold on cruise going that slow, I drove down the road on automatic at 25 miles per hour, steering around corners and laughing.

I felt that God had brought me that podcast from the Bear Creek Clinic using a friend at work, and it felt right to go there. Though an hour away, Medford was still part of "home," making it sound more comfortable. That's where I was going, covered by insurance or not. At least I was bound to get answers.

Sinking into an uncomfortable world, where my only relief was sleeping, reading the Bible, talking with Dave, or communicating on Facebook, I wondered where we were headed financially. I'd read about people losing their homes or spending

$100,000 out of pocket trying to get well from Lyme disease. We could lose the house we'd just built! We needed divine intervention for either my health or our finances or we could be facing bankruptcy.

Eleven

Occasionally, my symptoms would fade to bearable, like a mysterious wave of comfort, helping me to continue on with life. Maybe the coconut oil was helping a little. Or maybe God just touched me with reassurance once in a while. I had no idea.

When I started to think about the future, I got depressed, so I didn't think about it. This is easier when your brain is floating through a sea of forgetfulness, and you can't grasp a thought long enough to dwell on it. At times, I feared my thoughts were drifting away, and I would never get them back again. How much should I struggle to hold onto them? But I'd already tried. My entire day was a labor to focus on what I was doing, and failing. It was so much easier to let go and let God handle it, and I could remain at peace, knowing it was in His hands.

I'd read about people losing the ability to read or to drive when they had Lyme disease. This concerned me, because Dave couldn't drive and I spent most of my day reading or writing. Without these two things, I'd be lying around, staring at the scenery. Of course, with our view of Mt. Shasta and a lake, that wouldn't be so bad. But how would we get anywhere? The bus didn't come within two miles of us. Would Dave have to get a ride to church as well as a ride home? It bothered him to have to ask all the time. I wouldn't be able to work anymore if I couldn't drive. I hoped my condition would not go that far. Assuming it was Lyme, which I didn't know yet.

When *Healing Lyme* arrived, I was instantly hooked on reading it. The book gave me so much information that I was no longer sure I still needed to see the Lyme doctor. It was "Everything You Need to Know" to treat yourself for Lyme disease with natural remedies. Knowing the naturopathic doctor would be expensive, I wondered if I should cancel the appointment.

Certainly I could save a lot of money.

One week I couldn't wait to go and the next week I considered cancelling. What to do?

While trying to decide, I went down to the store and bought two of the three herbs that Buhner's book considered basic for healing Lyme disease: cat's claw and Japanese knotweed (resveratrol). The book said to start out slowly, so I only took one a day of each, increasing on the resveratrol to two or three per day. After all, I still didn't know if I had Lyme disease. But that was the beauty of using herbs. As with any food, they wouldn't hurt me unless I was allergic to them, and that was rare.

I was supposed to get copies of my lab tests from our local hospital before going to the Bear Creek appointment. When I finally remembered and went to pick them up, I was crestfallen. My first Lyme test was negative, and it was a Western blot antibody test, not the basic initial test recommended by the CDC. The Western blot was the more reliable test, wasn't it? It was also negative on all ten bands out of ten. Could that happen if I had Lyme?

What if it wasn't Lyme disease I had? I'd been so convinced that it was. Doctors often think it silly or even dangerous to diagnose yourself. I could be away off track.

One week after starting the herbs, I had a particularly difficult day at work, where I was on my feet longer, scanning some large drawings. So much pain and tingling surged through my body that I thought I would have to tell my boss I couldn't do that activity again, unless he wanted me to go home early, sick. My stomach hurt from too much pain reliever, and I wondered if I was getting an ulcer.

After going home and eating lunch, I went to bed for a nap. An hour or so later, the phone rang. Dave came into the bedroom and woke me up. It was a lady from the Bear Creek Clinic, calling because they had a cancellation and could fit me in! They said I could come up the next morning. The appointment was five weeks early, so I took that as a sign I should go. My bad, painful day had convinced me that I would not do very well on my own. I needed help.

Hoping I'd be able to drive up there, I endured the trip the best I could. I wanted David with me, as usual. I could lean on him when walking around, and he could carry things for me. Plus, we needed to buy things in Medford, where everything was cheaper, and I needed Dave to go inside the stores. I couldn't see myself walking around that much. My legs were so weak. In fact, when we parked and went to cross the street at the clinic, I wasn't able to "hurry" ahead when some cars were coming. My legs simply wouldn't go any faster.

The clinic looked like a house on the outside, but the inside was busy, with several doctors and office workers walking through the hallways. The walls were lined with shelves of bottled natural and herbal products, and one special shelf contained hundreds of tinctures with eye droppers.

What was I getting into? I was now in the hands of natural medicine and God. No going back now!

Twelve

Not knowing what to expect of Dr. Cory, Dave and I were both impressed with his knowledge and manner. I'd read that a licensed naturopathic doctor (an ND) is required to get a doctorate degree in medical school, plus learn all the herbal remedies and various natural protocols in addition to regular medical training. They just approach medical treatment from a more natural point of view.

Although my brain was wafting in and out of focus as usual, I managed to stay with it mentally during most of the ninety-minute consultation. Dr. Cory looked over my symptom list and asked questions related to Lyme disease that I expected. However, there was one line of questioning that I had not anticipated— a possible fungal infection.

I'd been exposed to mold for years in the old mobile home we lived in and at a previous job, and I knew I was allergic to the type of mold that grew in leaky walls. A couple of $250 tests would show up any issues, and of course I wanted to put off such expensive testing and focus on whether I had Lyme disease. Dr. Cory was going to test me for Lyme but he told me that he'd seen his Lyme patients struggle to get well if they had a mold toxin and did not take care of it. So I agreed.

Asking about the Western blot test I'd already had done, I wanted to know if it could show all ten bands negative if I had Lyme. He said yes and the fact that I'd started some of the herbal protocol might have brought the bugs out of hiding for the new test. I was glad I'd started the herbs at home ahead of time. Another blood draw was done to send for more Lyme testing.

At the end of the consultation, the doctor wrote out a bunch of instructions and lined up several bottles full of concoctions and a tincture specific to Lyme disease called "A-L" for Anti-Lyme. Even with no positive test in sight, I could tell this LLMD must think I had Lyme. He also added his own blend of "Lyme Ointment" to rub on especially painful areas, like my back and neck. He instructed Dave to rub it into my back when he did any massage.

Dr. Cory and his staff tried to arrange the paperwork in a way that might get my insurance to pay something, if possible. Feeling rather out of it, I hobbled out to the reception desk, where everything was rung up, except for a couple of tests, both of which we were all hoping would be covered by my insurance. It came to several hundred dollars, including the second appointment.

Worried, Dave pointed out the large total when he handed me the *American Express* receipt. I just shrugged. "What can I do about it now?" I whispered, not telling him that I had a feeling my insurance wouldn't pay anything for the lab tests either, whether they were in California or not. I knew I might be yet another example of a financially floundering Lyme victim, but at least I wouldn't have to buy my own antibiotics or get them in IV form. Before I discovered the naturopathic route, I thought we might lose everything we had trying to pay for treatment, because insurance doesn't typically pay for any treatment past a certain amount of time, including antibiotics. The CDC doesn't recommend it so the insurance companies won't pay for it. Several hundred dollars didn't sound like much in comparison to losing everything.

This new world of naturopathic medicine was the way I'd been led, and it was the way I'd followed. Right or not, I was getting treatment of some kind for my debilitating illness, and I felt it was certainly worth the money. I'd spent more than this in copayments trying to get help for my chronic cough in 2004 and 2005, and my current illness was far more serious.

After the miserable drive home from the doctor visit, I went straight to bed, wiped out from the trip and stress. When I got up, I set all the new bottles of herbs in front of me on our large coffee table and picked up the prescription list. Overwhelmed with all the new supplements, I picked up one jar at a time to examine it and the schedule. Most were indicated at meal times, but one had to be taken apart from meals twice a day, another had to be taken right before I ate, and yet another right after.

How am I going to do this with an inferior memory?

A spreadsheet was the answer! My favorite organization program awaited my command, so I created a chart, where I could check off pills as I took them.

Feeling a bit more organized, I opened the jars and sniffed. Most didn't have a smell, or they had a vague earthy aroma. The yellow curcumin smelled good to me, since I like curry. The doctor said this was to increase circulation and decrease inflammation. I was to avoid most pain relievers, but that was okay. I'd thought they were putting holes in my stomach anyway.

Another herbal blend was *HR-Stamina*, with a long list of ingredients I didn't recognize. I was supposed to take those in the morning only or it could keep me awake.

For heartburn, I had HCL betaine to take before a meal and a pepsin enzyme blend to take after. Taking an acid of any kind sounded terrible, but the doctor said heartburn was often caused by not enough stomach acid. He said my indigestion might clear up on its own eventually. I'd read about this kind of treatment before but was too afraid to try it.

Taking one HCL per meal, I was to increase to two per meal the next day and so on up to five per meal, until I felt a warm glow in my belly, then cut back to the dose from the day before. I wasn't in the mood to work on digestion with all my other symptoms, since taking an antacid at bedtime was easier. But I decided to try it anyway. When the warm glow hit the second day, I went back to one per meal.

The doctor said to increase the cat's claw up to three grams a day. I'd been only taking about 15% of that amount, so I was ready to see some action. Along with the resveratrol and my regular vitamins and meds morning and evening, I had a good-size collection.

Since the doctor had said it could be a mold toxin causing similar symptoms, I looked that up online. Sure enough, a mold infection could cause the fatigue, joint pain, and even the neurological symptoms I was having. Getting rid of it sounded terrible though— a very annoying diet with few carbohydrates, plus more pills or tinctures to take, most likely. I didn't want to think about it yet, but I'd already started to cut back on carbs to lose weight, so I figured it wouldn't be such a drastic change when the time came. Some NDs online recommended a similar diet for Lyme disease, so it couldn't hurt to start making a diet transition.

My next appointment wasn't for another six weeks. During that time, I'd have that same question going through my head, over and over: What if it wasn't Lyme disease?

Thirteen

A couple of years back, I'd wanted to cut back on so many pills. My vitamin B12 deficiency proved that a bad idea. But I'd been having trouble trying to remember the d-ribose powder I drank twice a day, for better muscle recovery due to my fibromyalgia. Trying to get down a lot more supplements wouldn't be easy.

That first evening, I took my large handful of pills and one drop of tincture at bedtime. Dave rubbed the new ointment on my back and neck, and I was amazed at how fast it worked. The pain just faded away, and I slept like a log. Was that because the ointment chased the Lyme bugs away from my spine? That seemed too bizarre to be true. Whatever was going on, I was impressed.

The next morning was Saturday, and I woke with a lot of "activity" in my left leg. That side had given me the most trouble during my illness, with numbness and tingling in various places. My left foot had ached for months, and I'd had to rub it often. It now quivered with a comfortable warmth, as though something soothing had been injected into my veins.

Increased circulation indeed! That was fast.

More strange sensations came over me during the day. My forehead above my right eye quivered a couple of times, like the left foot had. It was encouraging, because I figured the herbs were working in my body, and even in my head. When you think your body has been invaded with a stubborn bug, you are ready to drive it out any way you can. I'd read that some people ingest colloidal silver or take huge doses of various herbs to get rid of their Lyme disease on their own. Some are successful, but others end up sicker for quite a while.

The anti-Lyme liquid tincture sported a label with tiny writing I could not read without a magnifying glass. I wondered what was in the mysterious dark liquid as I put that first drop in water. It tasted like some kind of spicy unknown food, but at least it wasn't offensive. When I looked up the long names online, I found they were extracts of onion, garlic, cloves, black walnut, lemon and a few other plants.

The doctor had told me to start with one drop of the A-L tincture morning and evening, then increase to two drops, then three drops, and so on each day. He said at some point, I'd feel "really bad." This would be my cue to cut back to the previous day's dose and stick with it.

Great. I wondered what terrible thing would happen to me as each day dawned on this potent mixture. Vertigo? Worse fatigue? Inability to walk? Diarrhea? Vomiting? Bravely, I forged ahead, slowly increasing to the dreaded unknown dose of the future. On the other hand, maybe nothing would happen, because I didn't really have Lyme disease.

After six drops on the sixth morning, I felt a bit worse than usual but went to work anyway. Soon, I had pain in every joint. It was like the stuff had stirred the bugs out of every corner and they had rushed into new ones. The shooting pains had me saying "ouch" one minute and laughing the next at the weird pains and sensations. This continued all day. I decided this was feeling "really bad," so I cut back to 5 drops. I was so glad it was these oddball pains and not some other awful symptoms. Pain and I had been well-acquainted for years, and I usually could deal with intermittent pain better than certain other issues.

The treatment of bugs in the body, whether with antibiotics or herbs, often causes a *Herxheimer* reaction, commonly known as *herxing*. The *Chronic Illness Recovery* web site describes it this way: "Herxing is believed to occur when injured or dead bacteria release their endotoxins into the blood and tissues faster than the body can comfortably handle it. This provokes a sudden and exaggerated inflammatory response."[8]

---

[8] https://chronicillnessrecovery.org/index.php?option=com_content&view=article&id=161

So, now I had two more reasons to believe I had Lyme disease. The herbal treatment appeared to be causing a herxheimer reaction at the six-drop dose, and the Lyme specific ointment relieved the pain precisely where it was applied. The sharp pains finally ebbed in the evening of the six-drop dose of tincture, and I felt encouraged. If it was Lyme, my treatment was in progress and better yet, it was curable.

The next couple of weeks were a bit confusing. I had more energy, but was also more unsteady walking off and on. The pain in my neck seemed to just vanish. I had less pain in my jaw and less tingles and numbness on my left side. It was as though everything shifted around inside of me. Were the bugs migrating or what?

Sweating profusely for several days in a row, I thought it must be more than the hot weather or menopause. When I learned more about detoxification during herxing, I realized the sweating was a good thing. Apparently, detox helps the debris of dead bacteria in the body to move through the lymph nodes faster, speeding up recovery. I discovered too many detox methods online to try them all, but sweating occurs naturally. Was this yet another indication that it was Lyme disease?

About two weeks after I'd started the herbal protocol, I felt a lot worse again. Brain fog. Tingles. Pain. You name it, and it was all back. Now what? Finally it dawned on me that I had just increased the cat's claw to four grams the day before. The doctor had only prescribed up to three grams and I wasn't paying attention. I'd gone way over.

I was herxing from cat's claw, a primary Lyme disease herbal treatment! It must be Lyme!

Cat's claw is unlikely to cause any problem unless you're allergic to it, and I'd already been taking it long enough to know I wasn't. I cut back the herb to three grams and felt better by the next day. It was at this point that I was 99% certain I had Lyme disease. The increase and decrease of the Lyme targeting herb had affected me like clockwork, a strong indicator that this herb made the bugs inside me uncomfortable.

One day after a shaky walk around our local *WalMart* superstore, my legs felt like they might give way, even though I was leaning heavily on the cart. I had to turn the cart over to Dave, shuffle over to a bench by the door, and wait. It was too hot to sit out in the car. I didn't plan to go shopping again until I felt better.

Another day, my hip gave out completely for a second. All connections in my hip seemed to just disintegrate and then take hold again. A counter kept me from falling, but the episode scared me. I'd read about this kind of thing happening to people with Lyme disease. It happened again the next day, but not as bad.

I seriously considered buying a cane at this point, so I wouldn't fall. We still had a walker at home from Dave's recovery years ago, but I didn't feel emotionally ready for that. I didn't know how much pride I was hiding, until the thought of using a cane seriously bothered my self-esteem.

Holding off, I hoped the herbal treatment would start working soon enough to keep me free from assisted walking devices.

Fourteen

Three weeks after starting the new herbal regimen, my brain and body felt like I was pulling out of a long-term stupor. I had less pain, could walk better, and could hold a thought longer. My legs had strength in them, even if I did still walk funny at times. No cane needed after all!

My life looked like a movie running in reverse, as I noticed specific abilities returning in somewhat the same order they had left. Better thought processes alone were a reason to rejoice, but the sense of strength returning in my body added to the excitement. I felt at least 20-30% better! When all you've noticed is a downward trend for months, that is more than enough cause to celebrate.

Although it was a bit of two steps forward and one step backwards, the herbs began doing their job, and I was thanking God. That weekend, I had the energy to do some housework. Shopping at *WalMart* was okay again, and that was always a good test. My ability to hold myself upright had improved. I could sit up longer. Oh, and my heartburn went away.

Amazing!

For years I'd had pain in my back when washing dishes at the sink. But when washing some spinach at the kitchen sink one day, there was no pain. Leaning over for too long had likewise bothered my breathing for years, causing shortness of breath. When my garden started producing green beans, I leaned over for some time looking through the vines and picking them, without a problem. I wasn't sure if the herbs had chased the bugs away from certain spots or they just helped my joints limber up.

My worst symptoms had started in January, but I'd had other bad symptoms for ten years, like muscle pain that was diagnosed as FMS in 2004, which included some fatigue, a bit of tingling and nerve pain now and then, vertigo, and a horrible chronic cough that was so bad I pulled a muscle in my ribs once.

The weakness in my left arm had shown up at least five years before. I'd been scratching my left ear one day, but I could hardly move the fingers on my left hand in that position. It wasn't painful, it was more like paralysis.

All I'd ever been told was that I had FMS and allergies, so I had been taking a couple of different allergy pills, which kept my cough down a bit and my recurring vertigo at bay. I'd been treating my FMS muscle pain with d-ribose, a naturally sweet substance that doesn't affect blood sugar but helps muscles to recover faster. An anti-anxiety medication had also caused me to relax, helping my FMS and menopause symptoms, but I'd still felt like my health was a mess for at least thirty years.

Wondering how long ago I may have been bit by another tick and didn't notice, I remembered when the FMS first showed up. Didn't that and the fatigue hit me about the same time? FMS is a clinical diagnosis and there is no cure. Could it have been Lyme disease all along? I could have had Lyme for ten years and then been bit again more recently, adding a coinfection or just making everything worse.

The mold toxin I was being tested for could be the cause of the chronic cough and pretty much all the rest of the symptoms too, except maybe the tingling and numbness. I'd know soon what I had, because my appointment to get test results for the Lyme and mold toxin was only one week away.

For the next several days, my main problem was the fear that I didn't have Lyme disease. What would I do? Could I be helped at all? As much as it appeared like Lyme, there was always that one percent chance that it was something else, or some combination of things that produced the same symptoms. Trying to diagnose from symptoms was a common mistake, and I knew that. Yet, I'd read that Lyme was often a clinical diagnosis based on symptoms, due to unreliable testing.

At last the fateful morning arrived, and we headed back up to the Bear Creek Clinic. In Dr. Cory's office, Dave and I pulled our chairs up to his desk, so we could see the paperwork. Suspended in time as I awaited the pronouncement, I almost held my breath in anticipation of the outcome. Knowing that more negative results weren't always the end of the pursuit for Lyme diagnosis, I tried not to put so much weight into all the papers that the doctor spread out in front of us.

Not knowing what I was looking at on the papers, I listened for the verdict. Dr. Cory first pointed out that the same test given to me in my home town from a blood draw three weeks earlier than the new one was still negative, as was another test. So if he had only given these same tests as recommended by the CDC, I would still have only negative testing.

But the third test was positive! Not only was it positive as far as the Igenex Lab criteria where it was performed, it was positive per CDC standards! He said this meant it would automatically get reported to Public Health, where I'd be numbered in our County as another Lyme case. Some people went for years trying to get diagnosed, where I had only been trying for eight months. That lengthy search for a diagnosis alone was typical of Lyme disease.

I was one of those 50% false negative cases I'd read about, and the blood was drawn for the two tests only three weeks apart!

Thank God! How many people are able to rejoice in such a pronouncement? After all, late-stage Lyme is not easy to treat. But the positive test meant so many things to me, the best being that I'd already begun treatment that was working. I wouldn't get worse.

A positive Lyme test also meant I had been given the opportunity to share both my struggles and my recovery with others, using my own life and test-proven results. From what I'd experienced, the community in the area we lived in needed more education about Lyme disease, and I had a plan to spread the information needed.

At the beginning of Stephen Buhner's book *Healing Lyme*, his dedication reads: "For those people whose doctors told them it was all in their heads." That had encouraged me so much when I read it, as well as the content of the book. So had Brandilyn Collins' book *Over the Edge*, which so skillfully described what the baffling symptoms felt like to the person who had to struggle through them. Other books are on the market, but since Lyme is a rising epidemic, more good reading about Lyme disease is needed. I couldn't wait to write my own personal story.

Dr. Cory added a few more supplements to my protocol, some of which were for the mold toxins that were also found in my body, and he put me on a stricter diet to avoid mold and sugar. I was glad that I'd been able to stop a couple of the other supplements before taking on these new ones.

Excited, I went home knowing I was on my way back to health!

Fifteen

When I came back home, I had an appointment that I had been putting off, with my last doctor in Yreka. Debating back and forth, I wanted to cancel it now that I had a diagnosis, but I knew I needed to go in and show her my positive Lyme test and talk to her in person.

Nervous about what might happen, I waited for her to come into the exam room, almost biting my nails. What would she say? After the nurse checked my blood pressure and asked the usual questions, at last she came in the door, greeted me, and sat down.

Here goes... "I found out what was wrong with me," I said, pulling my test results out of my purse and trying not to anticipate trouble.

Startled, Doctor Three reached for the papers and examined them.

"You see," I went on in the silence that followed, "the naturopathic doctor I went to in Medford did a complete Lyme test panel. The IgG antibody test is still negative, just like the one you did for me, but the IgM is positive." I'd read that the two tests were targeted toward two different kinds of antibodies. I didn't know if she knew this, but I didn't presume to inform her. I barely knew what an antibody was. The two tests, one still negative and the other very positive, would cause her to investigate later on her own if she was curious. As a Physician's Assistant, she was probably still open to all the information she could gather. A long-term physician might be more likely to feel that his knowledge was complete and ignore the facts in front of him.

"Yes, I see." Doctor Three looked over the test results with a stunned expression, so I kept talking.

"I've read that the bacteria can encapsulate in the tissues and hide, so that the test comes back negative. That's probably what happened." There was a more scientific way to say this, something about a biofilm, but I hadn't learned enough about it to use it in a discussion. All the medical terminology tended to make my brain glaze over. Like the bacteria, I could hide too.

Doctor Three was listening to everything I told her, apparently fascinated. She told me she had almost gone into naturopathic medicine herself, so she liked the idea of using herbs. I shared a good web site for her to look at for more information, and she looked it up immediately. She asked if she could keep my list of herbs, because she had a couple of Lyme patients who were not getting better on antibiotics. Asking about the relieved pain in my back and neck, she wanted to know how to obtain Dr. Cory's Lyme Ointment as well.

Even better, Doctor Three said she was willing to work with Dr. Cory and order any tests my insurance would cover so that I didn't have to pay for everything myself. She was surprised that I no longer had heartburn, and she put pressure on my diaphragm to make sure it didn't bother me any more. She said she was glad I'd found someone to help but was sorry they hadn't been able to help me there.

Apology accepted.

Leaving the doctor's office that day, I was glad I'd decided to come. Hating confrontation, I never would have expected such a wonderful reaction from any local doctor. My plan for education in my hometown had started.

As I drove home, I thanked God over and over for helping me through the struggle, so I could help others. I had depended on Him, and He had brought what I needed to get me through. I'd hardly ever been depressed during my illness, though in so many ways I had good reason. I figured that was due to the many prayers going up for me and encouraging words that surrounded me with love and comfort.

Soon my problem was overdoing it too often. With a little energy in my system once again, I wanted to DO something. Unfortunately, the disease didn't agree with me, and when I started moving around a lot, I would suddenly get overly tired or have pain reminding me I was still sick and had a long way to go.

It's like when you get sick and you start feeling better, so you do too much then go through a relapse. Except the overall recovery runs over a much longer period of time than the usual viral or bacterial infection— weeks or even months of ups and downs. But as long as it was recovery, I wouldn't complain.

My mission is to educate as many people and health care professionals as possible about Lyme disease, hoping more people will find out where and how to get help so they don't end up worse. I figure if the Center of Disease Control thinks there are ten times more Lyme victims out there than are getting reported,[9] there must be a lot of people who need better testing and information. Lyme researchers feel the unreported number is much higher than the CDC thinks it is and that the bacteria can cause a chronic infection that lasts for months or even years.

I'm sure glad someone mentioned possible Lyme disease to me. Imagine what would have happened if my friend at work had not spoken up that day to share the podcast about the Bear Creek Clinic. I might still be wasting away, wondering what on earth was wrong with me.

---

[9] http://www.cdc.gov/media/releases/2013/p0819-lyme-disease.html

The sorrows of death encompassed me,
And the pains of hell got hold of me.
I found trouble and sorrow.
Then I called upon the name of the Lord,
"O Lord, I beseech Thee, deliver my soul."
Gracious is the Lord, and righteous;
Yes, our God is merciful.
The Lord preserves the simple.
I was brought low, and He helped me.
Return unto thy rest, O my soul,
For the Lord has dealt bountifully with thee.
For Thou hast delivered my soul from death,
My eyes from tears, and my feet from falling.
I will walk before the Lord in the land of the living.
I believed, therefore have I spoken:
"I was greatly afflicted."
Psalm 116:3-10

Resources

For more information about Lyme disease, http://www.ilads.org

To find a Lyme Literate doctor, http://www.lymediseaseassociation.org/index.php/doctors

For proven herbal treatment, http://buhnerhealinglyme.com

For symptoms of Lyme disease, http://canlyme.com/lyme-basics/symptoms

Other Books by Laurie Penner

In addition to the following books already published, Laurie has plans to write more short works like this one, about her other health experiences: chronic sinus infection and ten-year cough, hormones gone haywire, self-diagnosed celiac disease and food allergies, and taking care of her husband through his life-threatening conditions and situations. You can write to Laurie at writer7laurie@gmail.com, to find out when these new works will be coming out.

No Escape in Sight
An Inspirational Romance/Mystery Novel

When Beth Robertson's rebellious teenage girl disappears, the single mother imagines the worst. Has her daughter run away with some man? Former private investigator Luke Sanders offers to help, introducing to Beth a gentle but firm relationship that was unfamiliar to her during her previous marriage to an abusive alcoholic. Beth reluctantly befriends this unchurched man who has a good lead to find Emily and who obviously likes her. Beth and her twelve-year-old daughter Bonnie join Luke as he travels to Southern California, where the three search for clues and work together on a case that turns into an urgent race against time. When Luke's strikingly beautiful former girlfriend shows up to claim back Luke's attention, Beth's admiration of Luke falters. However, she is forced to endure Marlena's presence during the search. Relying on her faith in God to help her, Beth works through the complications until she can find Emily and get back to a normal life. As she tries to back away from any deeper relationship with Luke, Beth quickly realizes she is heading into yet another painful relationship from which there is no escape.

Mark of Love
An Inspirational Romance/Mystery Novel

Hidden away from the world by her mother because of a mark on her face, Amy Kramer lives in the shadow of her beautiful older sister. Suddenly forced by her mother to find a job when she is nineteen, Amy discovers that most of the world is unforgiving to someone who is so different in appearance. When she meets good-looking Zach Anderson, who works where she hopes to get a job, Amy can't help falling for his caring and friendly manner. But how can she hope to be happy, knowing that her sister is a more compatible and attractive mate for this man, especially when he obviously comes to the same conclusion?

Secrets of Gwenla
An Allegory

Breaking through fear and tradition.... Dealing with corrupt officials.... Struggling to understand the truth.... Julyiah must reveal the truth in time, or all will be lost!

Imagine living in two worlds at the same time—the physical one around you and another one inside you that no one else can see. Follow Julyiah as she searches for Gwenla's Book of Secrets and goes through her process of "Understanding," where anything can happen. In her world, some hearts dwell in cozy, peaceful places, while others are assaulted by fearsome powers.

Like their ancestors before them, Julyiah and her people remain locked away in their secret valley for 400 years, with none going in or out. Special rocks provide natural light and heat, as well as workable metals and building materials. Plenty of water allows them to grow crops and raise herds.

When Gwenla led the original group to safety 400 years ago, she also foresaw the future. Unable to safely pass on what she knew before she died, Gwenla wrote down her knowledge in riddles and hid them, so that only those who sought the truth would understand. Julyiah's adventurous heart wants to understand Gwenla's secrets, but when pressing to know the truth, Julyiah sees wonderful places outside the walls and hears forbidden music, disrupting her world and relationships.

In spite of several obstructions and evil forces trying to stop her, Julyiah discovers the truth and realizes she alone has the answer that will free the valley from deception. Yet her friends need urgent rescue as well. Can she accomplish both missions at the same time?

In a whirlwind of twists and turns that involve a severe time crunch, Julyiah must make connections from one end of the valley to the other, or she and those she loves will die, and the Secrets of Gwenla will remain hidden for all time.

Secrets Revealed
The Symbolism used in the Secrets of Gwenla

Mysterious, fantasy-style features surround Julyiah's special mission in Secrets of Gwenla. What do the spiritual symbols mean? Find symbols in the Bible that you've never seen before, in this little book.